This is not designed to be a 400 page guide…we want to give you the 10 most important secrets in 15 pages…

The definitive Quick-Start Guide on how to eliminate bad breath in 30 minutes

Table of Contents,

Chapter 9: Home Remedies for Bad Breath

 Chapter 10.Understanding the Various Types of Bad Breath Home Treatment

Chapter 11.   Stop Bad Breath and Be Happy

Dedication,

This book is especially dedicated to my dear mother and to all of my instructors. Please pray that Allah blesses them abundantly, and please accept my sincere gratitude on behalf of everyone who reads this lovely book.

Introductions

Introducing the ground-breaking How to get rid of bad breath in 30 minutes, the ultimate quick-start guide, and the best way to elevate your mouth. With the help of this outstanding book, you may easily provide a significant amount of fresh target to your body, ensuring maximum exposure and improved health.

The getting rid of bad breath was expertly crafted and supported by years of industry experience. It makes use of cutting-edge algorithms and techniques to produce an unstoppable wave of fresh good fragrance. Say goodbye to the struggle of trying to solve your problems; our books will take care of it for you by bringing you a steady stream of interested visitors or friends who want to interact with you.

With the help of this book, realize your full potential. You can increase your audience, broaden your network of health contacts, and finally take control of your health thanks to this inspiring book. As this book easily interacts with your ongoing, sound health activities to ensure maximum impact every day, you may watch as your health rates rise.

But don't just take our word for it; the how to get rid of bad breath in 30 minute has helped numerous people with astounding success. This is the best quick-start guide available. furthermore you joined.

Chapter 1:

How Not to Become a Victim of the Bad Breath Disease

You wouldn't want to experience the shame that comes with having foul breath, would you? We do, after all. And because of this, we always strive to maintain clean mouths and fresh breath. Yes, maintaining good oral hygiene is essential to preventing bad breath. Guess what, though? To combat anaerobic bacteria, an oral regimen alone is insufficient. To be prepared for foul breath when it occurs, you must have a thorough understanding of this ailment. Yes, poor breath disease can occasionally manifest. And that's what you ought to be ready for.

You must first understand the true nature of the ailment known as foul breath. You may discover comprehensive information about halitosis, or what is more popularly known as foul breath, in a variety of online sources.

You can look for information about dental health online, read some books and magazines, or just ask your dentist directly. You will learn about the various causes that can create foul breath in addition to finding out facts about bad breath.

So who or what is to blame? These are a few:

* Tooth decay — If one or more of your teeth are decayed, you should anticipate having bad breath.

* Periodontal disease, sometimes referred to as gum disease; if you have gum disease, you are probably going to have poor breath.

* Plaque – there is a great likelihood that you will have bad breath if you have plaque or even a few food particles between your teeth.

* Tonsil or Throat Infection — certain issues in the throat are also known to create foul breath. We require saliva to wash out the meals in our mouths, but if you have dry mouth, these food particles will linger there and cause unpleasant odor.

It is best to actually contact a dentist if you already suspect that you have bad breathThe best course of action will be suggested to you by your dentist. A prophylaxis is typically carried out to determine whether dental plague or food stagnation is to blame for poor breath. Now, if an oral cause cannot be found, you might need to visit additional clinics that focus on breath odor issues. Or perhaps you are simply overly attentive to your breathing and the issue is psychological.

But, what the heck? Actually, how you take care of yourself and maintain good oral hygiene will determine how fresh your breath is. You can do the following things to ensure that your breath always smells good:

* Use floss or other specialty brushes as directed by your dentist to ensure that difficult-to-reach areas in the mouth are fully cleaned. Simple brushing is insufficient to thoroughly clean the teeth and mouth. Clean your tongue. Dental professionals advise using tongue cleaners to clean your tongue all the way to the back, where odor-producing germs tend to live.

* Mouthwash it — It is advised to use mouthwash after meals or before bed if you can't brush.

* A healthy diet – consuming fiber, fresh veggies can help you always keep your mouth clean.

Drinking less coffee will also be beneficial.

⌐ Drink extra water; this will encourage your body to create more saliva, which is necessary to wash away food particles in your mouth.

Chapter 2: How to prevent bad breath

Ad breath is not a straightforward condition that you can simply brush off and ignore. Although significant dental and medical disorders are not always the result, it might nevertheless cause more problems than you anticipated. A condition like bad breath can make you feel self-conscious and cause you to lose confidence. The only thing it ever does is come out of your mouth, and the whiff makes the people you talk to close up cover their noses or step back a little. Accept it. Not only is it embarrassing, but it's also unsettling. This embarrassing situation may depress you mentally and emotionally.

Why does foul breath happen?

When food particles linger in the mouth, bad breath, or halitosis as it is medically referred to, develops. These include detritus on the tongue, in the mouth's lining, and between teeth. There are some bacteria that keep themselves occupied to stop the growth of harmful bacteria.

However, when you don't brush your teeth and mouth to remove these debris, harmful germs are attracted and quickly establish a colony inside. Bad bacteria spread substances that now give your breath a bad odor.

Another factor contributing to poor breath is a lack of water consumption. Because there is less moisture for the harmful germs to work on, dry mouth is where they love to live.

Additionally, smoking makes your breath smell terrible. And not just that. It can lead to the accumulation of tartar and plaque, which is another factor in bad breath.

Infections including tonsillitis, sinusitis, and other similar illnesses are another cause of bad breath.

Infections transport substances that are absorbed by the mouth and give breath an unpleasant odor. In addition to this, some medical diseases such kidney issues, diabetes, periodontitis, and others can cause halitosis.

Additionally, someone who uses prescription medications may also be at risk for developing halitosis.

There are several different prescription medications that, when taken orally, make breath smell awful.

How to Keep Breath Fresh

Bad breath is preventable. Regular oral and dental hygiene practices are one option you have.

A quick but efficient technique to stop the growth of the harmful bacteria that causes halitosis in your mouth is to brush and floss twice a day.

Mouthwash is also advised in order to completely clean your mouth and breath. The rinse removes any debris that may have been left on the tongue and mouth lining because brushing and flossing do not completely remove all of the debris from your mouth.

Additionally, scraping your tongue is a fantastic approach to stop the growth of harmful microorganisms.

By keeping your mouth wet throughout the day with water, you can keep these bacteria from proliferating and prevent the formation of harmful substances.

As soon as you experience symptoms, you must consult your doctor and dentist. Even if you maintain good oral hygiene, if your foul breath persists, there may be a problem with your medical condition. If so, your doctor or physician should make the diagnosis and administer the necessary care.

The first step to treating halitosis and regaining your confidence afterward is speaking with your dental hygienist. It is never easy to think about having bad breath. Take care of your own hygiene and visit your doctor frequently if you don't want to experience the negative effects it brings.

Bad Breath in Toddlers: Facts and Possibilities, Chapter 2a.

The growth of our children is just so incredible. You simply can't believe how large your once-small baby has become and how active he has become. You always want the best for your child since you're a mother, after all. You want him to be well-built, have brilliant eyes, and perhaps have pearly white teeth.

You undoubtedly desire your infant to always have baby fresh breath in addition to the latter.

Now, if you learn that your infant has terrible breath, you will undoubtedly be in a hurry. Yes, it is unexpected because the majority of people think that babies won't have foul breath. However, this is just typical. Yes, toddlers with terrible breath are common. Even though it is rare that they will consume pungent foods like garlic and onions, they could nonetheless have unpleasant breath.

The following are some things that can cause children to have bad breath:

Babies are more likely to have foul breath than adults because they sleep longer than adults, which reduces saliva production. Babies and toddlers also tend to have terrible breath since most of them breathe through their mouths most of the time. Why? Because breathing via the mouth will dry it out and encourage the growth of bacteria that produce odors. Things associated with newborns and toddlers, such as sucking thumbs or blankets, can also result in dry mouth.

You should take care of your toddler's mouth because they are still too young to understand the importance of good oral hygiene. What can you do, then, to stop kids from having foul breath? Here are a few examples:

e The greatest way to prevent bad breath in children is to practice good oral hygiene, such as the following;

Drinking enough of water, rinsing your mouth after meals, properly cleaning your tongue, and brushing and flossing your teeth as directed * A excellent strategy to keep your baby's breath fresh is to get adequate oral hygiene items for your child.

* Visit your child's pediatrician frequently. By doing this, you may ensure that your child never gets sick and never develops the type of illness that frequently results in foul breath.

The first skill you can teach your toddler is how to properly wash their teeth. This will guarantee that your child develops healthy oral habits at a young age, resulting in consistently fresh breath and a clean mouth. In addition, you can prevent your youngster from eating foods with strong scents and foods with a lot of sugar.

You can do your own study if you still need additional details about kids' terrible breath. The greatest method for you to do that is online. There are several websites online that offer instructions, advice, and tips regarding foul breath in kids. To get the specific tidbits of information you require, you can search these websites. But, you know what, the dental office is the best resource for information.

Consult your dentists for advice on the best ways to protect your young children from the inconveniences of foul breath and an unhealthy mouth.

Understanding Children's Bad Breath in Chapter 2b.

The children have the cleanest breath of all. But what would you say if your own child had this condition?

Although that's not supposed to be the case in a child's formative years, it also can't be avoided. If the youngster has nasal drip or is not being controlled in maintaining adequate dental hygiene, this will worsen. Additional oral problems can contribute to this syndrome. Here are a few reasons why your child may have bad breath even at this young age.

1. Bad dental hygiene. Young children have no concept of oral hygiene or any of the other sorts of hygiene that one should practice. Even if it requires them to complete it alone, you must assist them in comprehending its purpose and the reasons behind why they must do it frequently. To make it interesting for kids to practice oral hygiene on their own, you can swap up the brands and flavors of toothpaste.

decay in the teeth. Serious dental decay is one of the most common causes of bad breath in children. His breath smells just like this, so you can tell. It has the same rotting scent that his teeth do.

3.) A few ailments, such as acute and chronic sinusitis. These particular sinusitis kinds frequently result in nasal drips or discharges, either directly from the nose or via the mouth-nose connection, which is located at the top of the mouth. A child's mouth or breath may become contaminated by these drips, which will also contribute to his bad breath.

4. A Pharyngitis warning indication. Because of the bacterial illness he or she is experiencing, a child who has a nose, throat, or pharyngitis will undoubtedly have a terrible odor in their mouth.

5.)Allergies. Your child's poor breath may also be brought on by seasonal allergies. Some allergies can lead to postnasal drips, which, like sinusitis, can leave the mouth smelling awful. This is due to the bacterial illnesses that may also be responsible for these offensive scents.

6.) A thing that is rotting in the mouth or nose. It is dangerous to leave a child alone. Without you knowing it, he or she might put something in their mouth. This may be a maize kernel, a pea, or anything else that will make him or her laugh. They start to decompose, stink, and smell when they are kept in the nose or mouth for longer than a day. The child's breath will pick up this odor for a short while before it disappears completely.

When they are dealing with embarrassing situations like foul breath, children are quite likely to have the same challenges as adults. This is why it is crucial that you give the best advice you are able to. If they are practicing good oral hygiene as you instructed, have them checked frequently.

Don't let them skip any of these because it's for their own benefit and what they learn now will change as the years go by. You don't want them to experience unpleasant circumstances where their friends and family withdraw from them, do you?

Steps for Eliminating Bad Breath; Know What to Do. Chapter 3.

It's critical to get treatment for bad breath right away because it can ruin a romantic moment with your partner. Halitosis and bad breath can be avoided by maintaining good oral hygiene. This entails very frequent tooth brushing and cleansing. Additionally, flossing will be a huge assist in accomplishing the same.

It could be exceedingly challenging for your seatmate, family, or even friends to smell your breath. However, you may get it treated, prevented, or even self-test to see if you have it. Tips for diagnosing and treating foul breath are provided below:

1.) Licking your wrist is one of the simplest ways to determine if you have bad breath. Give it at least five seconds to dry. Once it has dried, smell it. What scent does it have to you? You smell like that when you breathe out, or more specifically, your breath does.

2.) If you are certain that your mouth smells unpleasant, you need to improve your dental hygiene.

While you don't have to go overboard, make sure you still exercise consistently. Better oral hygiene products, such as mouthwash and breath fresheners, will also encourage a better mouth odor.

The aforementioned scenario is a minor cause of halitosis. There are more severe instances of this oral ailment, which involves overcoming odor. This is distinguished by an extremely unpleasant odor that persists despite frequent tooth brushing. You'll still have that unpleasant odor in your mouth for a few minutes after brushing. If you are currently dealing with this, you need to get in touch with a reputable dental expert right away for assistance.

Bacteria that grow in the mouth, particularly in the back of the tongue, are typically the source of bad breath. The anterior, or frontmost, and posterior, or back, are the two parts that make up the tongue. On the tongue, mouth walls, and teeth, bacteria frequently gather. The tongue is where bacteria are most common. If you have this condition, you can also perform an effective self-test using the advice below:

1.) To do the test, obtain a spoon, preferably one made of metal. Scrabble the back of your tongue. If, after scraping, there is some white substance in the spoon, don't be concerned. That is perfectly normal and the purpose of the surgery.

2. Inhale the white matter's aroma. If it smells extremely foul, you can be certain that oral bacteria are residing in your rear and are the source of the foul smell.

3.) Maintain your usual dental hygiene routine while using a mouthwash or deodorizer that is more effective and has been proved to eliminate odors. Before going to sleep is the ideal time to use these resources.

4.) Clean your tongue towards the rear of your mouth using a tongue cleaner.

5.) Drink plenty of liquids, but try to limit your intake of alcohol and coffee because they often leave residues on your tongue that will make your condition worse.

Chronic Bad Breath: Know the Facts and Prevent It, Chapter 4.

Your social life may become persistently hampered by persistent bad breath. It may even keep you from making new acquaintances and forming new relationships. But how can you be certain that your halitosis is worse?

There are more options than you can count that won't put you in embarrassing circumstances.

There are also a few bodily cues to be cautious. Here are some pointers on how to recognize it:

1. The anterior and posterior halves of the tongue are separate structures.

The back of your tongue is called the posterior, while the front is considered the anterior. A white or yellow film that develops on your tongue frequently, especially on the back, is a sign that you may have bacteria of the Halitosis is already present. To scrape that area of your tongue, get a good metal or silver spoon.

The soft, white, or yellow substance you obtain as a result shouldn't bother you. It's not the most crucial or the major issue, and if it stinks that horrible, you undoubtedly have bad breath. Another method is to lick your wrist, which will dry in five seconds or less. Whatever it is that you smell, that is how you appear to others.

2.) The mouth shouldn't taste and smell that terrible at the same time. If you frequently experience that unpleasant taste in your mouth, you should be aware that this is the primary sign that you have extremely poor breath.

3.) When others withdraw when you are speaking, this is another sign that you have foul breath. This condition merely shows that you are a bad talker because you pollute the air, thus you should be conscious of it.

4.) There are some persons who are more outspoken or upfront about the fact that they have persistent bad breath. On the other side, other people are less direct and might just offer you candies, mints, or chewing gum.

5.) Losing friends or having people avoid talking to you or just being around you is another extremely good sign that you have chronic bad breath.

Social development is crucial for everyone. This is why you need to start treating your persistent foul breath right now. But how do you go about it? Additionally, there are a variety of techniques to both prevent and treat it. Below is a list of several for your consideration.

1. Maintain better dental hygiene. The trick is to perform it correctly and frequently. Don't just brush it off.

Use mouthwash and floss for even greater results.

2.) Drink lots of fluids, but refrain from consuming coffee or alcohol, as these beverages leave behind residues that may worsen your halitosis.

3. Consume fibrous foods, which are excellent for your dental and general health.

4.) Because fish, meat, and dairy products have such strong flavors, you should always wash your teeth, tongue, and gums after eating them.

5.) You should always conclude your routine of brushing your teeth by giving your tongue a special attention in the rear, where bacteria thrive.

Use these suggestions, and your therapy for persistent bad breath will undoubtedly change your life.

Do You Have The Signs of Bad Breath? is Chapter 5.

Are your coworkers beginning to gently avoid you? Do the individuals you are speaking with in front of notice when you are talking to them? Every time you talk, do they cover their mouths? If you answered yes to each of these questions, are you certain that these situations have caused you to lose confidence?

And it's unsettling, yes? You are aware that there is a problem with you.

You may be 100% correct if you assumed it was because you have foul breath, or halitosis, which is a condition where you have it. Those are the indications of poor breath in each of the circumstances stated above.

And if you don't take good care of it, those situations will happen more frequently.

You don't want that since it could lead to you having no friends at all. The difficulty with halitosis is that it can be difficult to determine whether you already have it. The reason is that you are unable to smell your own breath with your nose. Always, someone else must notice your terrible breath before you do.

Sometimes, foul breath can get so unbearably pungent that people can smell it from a considerable distance away.

Halitosis can have a variety of reasons.

Bad breath sufferers frequently struggle to maintain good oral and dental hygiene. Food and drink residue from improper tooth cleaning and flossing is left between the teeth and on the mouth's lining. Your breath smells terrible because the particles feed harmful bacteria.

Another factor that contributes to halitosis is a dry mouth. When people don't frequently moisten their mouths by drinking a lot of water, internal alterations take place. First, the saliva and germs in the mouth that have previously gathered become considerably more concentrated. The acid or base balance of saliva tends to change, making it a popular breeding site for harmful bacteria. The shifting of the acid or base balance evaporates into the air while your mouth remains dry, resulting in that revolting bad breath.

When you can see a yellow or white film on your tongue, you also have terrible breath. This occurs when nasal mucus leaks into the tongue's surface areas. When the nasal mucus, saliva, and mouth lining combine, the harmful bacteria in the mucous and its foul odor cause your breath to become foul-smelling as well. In most cases, removing the tongue's film with a brush or scraper will not solve the issue. To address the root of the issue, a treatment must be sought.

Bad breath symptoms might also affect those who are taking drugs. Taking medication frequently leads in unpleasant tastes like bitter, metallic, and sour tastes. Additionally, this leads to the growth of harmful germs, which results in bad breath. Bad tastes can also be reported in conjunction with tonsillitis, sinus discharge, dental restorations that have been damaged, and tooth diseases. Each of these circumstances results in a decrease in salivation, which contributes to bad breath.

You already have the symptoms of bad breath if brushing, flossing, and mouthwashing are ineffective at treating your halitosis. There is no better course of action in this regard than to see your dentist or doctor to make sure the issue is properly identified and addressed.

Chapter 6: A Variety of Breath Problems

It's intriguing to realize that your mouth is home to millions of different types of bacteria. You probably believed that these germs were the root of foul breath. Despite the fact that they are frequently blamed for the embarrassing mouth condition, not all of them are genuinely unpleasant. The majority of them work assiduously to maintain your mouth's health by assisting with food digestion and preventing harmful germs from growing.

What then are the reasons of foul breath if it is not bacteria?

Bad breath is a condition that gives off a bad odor, can be unpleasant, and can cause psychological and emotional setbacks for the person who has it. It is not caused by all of the bacteria in the mouth, but some conditions can make good bacteria turn bad and produce substances with unpleasant odors. When food and drink particles interact with saliva, they create harmful bacteria, especially if oral hygiene is not practiced.

Here are a few typical reasons why people develop bad breath:

Due to dry mouth, it is advised that you drink enough of water to keep your mouth wet and prevent germs from producing harmful substances. Although the saliva in the mouth is thought to be the natural cleaning agent, if it were to get dry, plaque would likely have a better chance of accumulating on the teeth. When the germs in the oral area are fed into this plaque, bad breath eventually results. Then, throughout the day, drink lots of water to keep your mouth and breath clean.

Poor oral hygiene makes it simple for harmful germs to assemble in your mouth if you don't maintain good oral hygiene. Then, plaque and tartar form, destroying not just your teeth but also your breath. The ideal places for these germs to grow are plaque and tartar, therefore it's critical that you practice good dental hygiene, which includes routinely brushing, flossing, and occasionally mouth washing. If plaque and tartar have already accumulated, a trained dentist should be consulted for professional care and treatment to prevent further spread.

Even when you maintain good dental hygiene and keep your mouth hydrated, sinus issues can occasionally cause your breath to still smell bad. In this instance, a specific medical ailment, in particular a sinus disease, may have led to this. You have terrible breath as a result of excess mucus building up on your tongue. Since mucus already has a poor odor, when it touches the tongue and remains, it encourages the growth of germs that lead to bad breath. It is best to visit a doctor if you have a sinus disease so they can prescribe the right medications.

Similar to sinus infection, other infections can also result in bad breath, therefore it's crucial to speak with your doctor to make sure they are correctly treated. Halitosis, or just bad breath, can be prevented and cured if the causes are identified and addressed.

You can avoid the humiliation that comes with having bad breath by practicing good dental hygiene, drinking plenty of water, treating certain medical issues properly, and obtaining frequent medical examinations.

Chapter 7: Numerous Remedies for Bad Breath

Who desires foul breath? No, I assume. You would never imagine having such an issue because you don't want others to keep their distance when speaking with you. Sad to say, some people will even try to avoid speaking to you directly. As soon as you realize you have bad breath, you should research the many foul breath remedies.

Halitosis, generally known as bad breath, can undoubtedly hinder your success both personally and professionally. It's a good thing that this issue can be fixed. In fact, according to the Center for Breath Treatment, there is now a very successful treatment for Americans who have this ailment. To prevent this problem from affecting your immediate family and close acquaintances, you should first be aware of its causes.

Causes of Bad Breath * Dental Decay and Ill Gums

The most frequent reason for bad breath is this. The gums will develop abscesses filled with foul-smelling pus when the roots of your teeth begin to deteriorate, which will lead to bad breath. And did you know that even the smallest gaps in your teeth can serve as a breeding environment for microbes that cause bad breath?

* issues with the throat, nose, and respiratory system

You did read that correctly. The health of your respiratory system, particularly your nose, throat, and respiratory tract, has an impact on how you breathe. Your breath smells bad if you have sinusitis, chronic gastritis, chronic tonsillitis, or lung conditions. Additionally, digestive disorders, increased constipation, and intestinal sluggishness can all lead to episodes of bad breath.

Natural Remedies for Bad Breath * Fenugreek therapy

The most effective at-home treatment for halitosis is fenugreek usage. To solve this issue, daily consumption of the tea derived from the seeds of this vegetable is required. The following is how to make this tea: Put one teaspoon of seeds in half a liter of cold water, and simmer it for fifteen minutes on a low flame. To make a tea, strain it.

Treatment for Avocado Halitosis

Another successful treatment for foul breath is the avocado fruit. It is significantly more efficient than other mouthwashes and remedies for foul breath. Such fruit effectively reduces intestinal putrefaction, which is a frequent source of bad breath. Guava Breath Freshener

Guavas that are still green are also useful for curing halitosis since they contain the acids malic, phosphoric, tanic, and oxalic. Additionally, it contains calcium, oxalate, and manganese. The guava fruit is a great tonic for gums and teeth thanks to these acids and nutrients. Chewing tender guava leaves can also halt bleeding from the gums and teeth.

* Parsley Therapy

One of the many remedies for foul breath is parsley, which is created by boiling two cups of water with two to three whole cloves and finely chopped parsley. Only a quarter teaspoon of ground cloves will do if you use them. Stir this mixture sporadically while it cools. Use it as a gargle several times a day after straining.

Even while these various remedies for bad breath work, you shouldn't overlook the easy techniques to maintain a reasonable amount of breath odor. Remember to brush and floss your teeth at least twice daily, preferably right before night. To remove meat fragments, use a toothpick. A dentist needs to take care of your decaying teeth and infected gums, however.

Chapter 8: Use Bad Breath Medicines To Treat The Symptoms.

You'll probably feel rejected if individuals run away from you when you try to strike up a discussion, thinking that they don't want you. This can be a terrible experience, especially if it occurs more than once, perhaps even more than twice. Instead of moping around, check yourself since you might have halitosis, or just foul breath. The truth is that most individuals find it intolerable when they smell someone else's foul breath.

It's funny how sometimes people can tolerate speaking with physically unclean people, but it is nearly impossible to continue a conversation with someone who exhales foul air. So, if you've been feeling rejected, ask yourself if you actually do have that feeling. If you do, don't complain about it; instead, look for bad breath remedies to treat it and prevent a repeat of the situation.

It's crucial to keep in mind that there are no miraculous drugs that will instantly cure your ailment when looking for bad breath remedies. First and foremost, you must identify the cause of your foul breath before purchasing an over-the-counter medication. There are medications for foul breath available, but they are actually provided in various ways. Not every one of these approaches is the best choice for your situation.

Therefore, identify the true cause of your halitosis before spending money on medications. There are many different causes of halitosis, and the one you have will largely determine how you should be treated.

So, for instance, if poor oral hygiene is the cause of your bad breath, all you need to do is make sure to remedy this mistake and keep up with it. But if your illness is more severe than that, you need to find another solution. For instance, before using bad breath medications, you must first treat any related medical disorders, such as sinusitis, tonsillitis, and others.

Meanwhile, severe foul breath symptoms can be treated with herbs, minerals, and other natural items. Many people have been depending on the wonders of natural resources since they not only efficiently treat problems with bad breath, but also because they contain therapeutic natural ingredients that make them perfect to promote good physical condition and a healthy mouth. Depending on the true cause of your halitosis disease, additional types of bad breath medications may be suggested if you contact a dental professional or medical specialist.

No matter what anti-bad breath medications are recommended, it's crucial to maintain good dental hygiene in addition to taking the prescription. Among the most crucial good habits to adopt to prevent bad breath are brushing, flossing, mouthwashing, avoiding spicy foods, and taking care of your physical health.

Not only should you smile more frequently if your mouth and breath are in good health, but you should also feel more confident when speaking in front of an audience. You'll discover that it's also a quality that most people would prefer in a conversation partner rather than having to endure a terrible case of bad breath coming from the other person.

A good breath would never interfere with your social life, making it much easier and happier overall.

Chapter9: Home Remedies for Bad Breath

Ever felt uncomfortable in front of others because of the smell of your breath? Or has it caused you to feel a little bit less confident and less inclined to interact with people? These are merely the initial, visible affects of having poor breath. Halitosis is the medical word for bad breath.

The saliva of a person should smell distinct. However, the food consumed and the bacteria that produce a strong odor in the saliva will alter this fragrance. However, it's not the fragrance of the saliva itself that contributes to foul breath. The bacteria that live in the tongue's lining and other areas of the mouth are what give someone terrible breath.

But from where did these microorganisms originate? Ironically, the bacteria are leftovers from the food that people eat. In a straightforward experiment, food that is not eaten at the table will eventually go bad. The germs are by-products of the spoiled food remnants that individuals consumed. Because human saliva contains a digestive ingredient, the decay of food remnants happens even more quickly.

Halitosis is neither a disease or a fatal ailment, which is a good thing. It's merely a sanitary issue. Halitosis, however, can cause troubles in the mouth, such as gum and throat issues among others, if it is not appropriately addressed and treated. In addition to this implication, you run the risk of alienating some friends or making headlines.

Since halitosis is essentially a hygienic issue, the main thing one can do to eradicate or resolve it is to promote cleanliness. It is advisable to regularly brush your teeth and to clean your tongue and other oral tissues. When foul breath is not eliminated or returns after a few hours, attempt to use these straightforward, at-home solutions.

1.) Check for damaged teeth. Since the germs prefer to live in areas of the mouth that are not frequently cleansed by regular brushing, it is preferable to have the tooth pulled rather than repaired. 2.) Take into consideration mouth rinse — mouth rinse is a very powerful mouth cleanser. For thorough operations, you may inquire with your dentist about this. They are designed specifically to attack oral bacteria, which may survive in the tiniest spaces in the mouth. You can pick from a wide variety of brands and tastes when purchasing this product.

3.) Drink lots of water. This will not only help you flush toxins from your body, but it will also keep your mouth moist, which increases saliva production and forces contaminated saliva into the body's waste channels. Drinking more water will help you flush food debris from your mouth and into your intestines, which will lessen the likelihood that you'll get foul breath.

4.) Chew gum—this is a short-term solution. You can choose to chew gum whenever you feel that your mouth is already dry and you do not have access to water. Gums with a cinnamon flavor are thought to have odor-removal abilities that assist prevent bad breath. Gums with flavors like spearmint and eucalyptus are also an option.

5.) Give up smoking; studies have shown that foul breath is one of the side effects of smoking. This is because nicotine and tar can build up in the tongue's lining, which can result in unpleasant mouth odor.

Just keep in mind that halitosis isn't exactly an illness. In this case, hygiene is key. This will undoubtedly prevent foul breath.

Chapter 10: Understand the Various Home Remedies for Bad Breath

The most embarrassing oral condition a person can have is undoubtedly bad breath, often known as halitosis. Your work life as well as your own personal being will be affected by this dental problem. Therefore, it's crucial to get treatment as soon as you realize you have it in your mouth. And if you really feel uncomfortable disclosing this extremely private sanitary condition, you may just use the at-home cure for bad breath designed for those who have it but are reluctant to disclose it, even to dental specialists. However, before receiving therapy, you must confirm that you actually possess it by following these candid advice:

1.) Convince yourself that your foul breath is real in order to avoid overreacting or practicing excessive oral hygiene. Your wrist will dry in about five seconds after you lick it. then take a whiff. What scent does it have to you? It smells exactly the same to other people as your breath does.

2.) It's time to assess how awful your bad breath is if you do. Grab a silver or metal spoon, and use it to scrape the back of your tongue. By the way, the anterior of your tongue is the front portion, and the posterior is the back. The halitosis bacteria are most prevalent in the posterior. After scraping, smell the residue that is still in the spoon. This time, how does it smell to you? It's unfortunate that you have persistent foul breath if it's worse than you thought!

Here is a list of effective home remedies you can take to treat yourself in the comfort of your own home now that you are aware of the quantity of foul breath you will be experiencing:

enhancing your oral hygiene practices. This time, using a toothbrush alone is not sufficient; you also need to use a mouthwash and deodorizer. Do this consistently and correctly.

2.) You must also brush your tongue from the back toward the tip.

3.) Ensure that you brush your teeth after consuming dairy products, meats, and fish. Alternatively, if a toothbrush is not accessible, gurgle mouthwash.

4.) Be sure to drink plenty of fluids, but avoid coffee and alcohol because they can make your dental condition worse.

Eat a diet rich in fiber. These foods are extremely safe for your oral health.

6. Have your children or nieces and nephews take a breathalyzer test. Ultimately, they won't care if you come up with inventive ways to accomplish it. Making fun of it or simply comparing your odours is among the best methods. Or, if even children make you feel that testing your breath will make you appear foolish, you might use the methods outlined above to monitor your progress.

If you are happy with how things are going, don't be content and resume your lax dental hygiene habits. Continue putting what you've learned into practice, and you'll soon discover that the persistent foul breath you once had is completely gone. Knowing no one knew you discussed it in the privacy of your house will make it even more pleasant.

Because you never formally acknowledged having it, nobody will even think you once did.

Chapter 11: Stop Breathing Badly and Smile

When you speak to somebody, do they move away from you? Verify your breathing. Perhaps they simply can't stand the smell. If you have foul breath, it's easy to detect.

All you have to do to smell something is blow on a handkerchief or your palm. If it smells unpleasant, you had best take action right once to stop bad breath!

You are aware that having foul breath doesn't help you. In addition to ruining your chances of success in both your personal and professional life, it will make people shun you. You should now look for techniques, even natural ones, to stop foul breath if it doesn't sound that great to you.

Tips to Get Rid of Bad Breath: Floss and Brush Your Teeth Frequently

The simplest yet most effective techniques to combat bad breath are brushing and flossing. Keep in mind that the germs on our teeth and gums are the main source of bad breath. These bacteria multiply on food particles lodged between teeth and release volatile sulfur compounds that give you sour breath. frequent tongue cleaning

Do you know that some of the germs that cause bad breath hide in your tongue's crevices? Since the majority of these bacteria cannot survive in the presence of oxygen, they prefer your mouth as their refuge since it allows them to conceal themselves on food particles and beneath a barrier of proteins and mucus. Get a tongue cleaner and clean your tongue of this layer and the bacteria that live beneath it to stop this. Don't forget to brush the back of your tongue. boost your water intake

The ideal environment for odor-producing bacteria is a dry mouth. Saliva helps to keep the mouth moist and cleans away food particles, which helps to dissolve volatile sulfur compounds. However, we engage in behaviors that decrease salivation and result in a dry mouth. These include: - Taking prescribed medication - Talking excessively - Exercising - Drinking alcohol - Dieting - Smoking

How then can you enhance saliva production? Simple. Simply drink a lot of water. By doing so, food particles are removed and your mouth becomes moist, making it less welcoming to bacteria that cause odors.

Eat Only Sugar-Free Gums

After eating, if you are unable to brush your teeth, chew some sugarless gum. This cleans your teeth and encourages salivation. * Gargle with chlorine dioxide Mouthwashes

Chlorine dioxide-containing mouthwashes are the best for fighting foul breath. Such a chemical specifically targets the volatile sulfur molecules that give your breath a bad odor. Look for indications of dental issues

Make sure you don't have periodontal disease because there are perfect places for bacteria that cause odors to hide. The following are some indicators of periodontal disease: - Swollen gums

- Pain when biting - Sensitive or loose teeth - Puss around the teeth - Sensitive and bleeding gums.

  At least once per year, visit the dentist.

Adults should go to the dentist at least once a year to have their teeth examined. The dentist is aware of the warning indications of dental issues, therefore you will be given advice on how to prevent them. Since they can identify abscesses, impacted teeth, periodontal disease, and other issues causing bad breath, your dentist is also the best person to consult about it.

So, stop bad breath by implementing these suggestions. These suggestions are straightforward and simple to implement, yet they have a significant impact on removing the offensive odor from your mouth.

Conclusions

Bad breath can be a short-term or chronic condition. Regardless matter which of these two you have it is Not a good story. Imagine how embarrassing it will be to have this condition. Not to mention that the smell may cause people to avoid talking to you. It is fortunate that you do not have this issue because of this.

Be cautious though, as there are numerous causes of bad breath. Having a thorough understanding of the various factors that contribute to bad breath is the best defense against it. The most typical causes of bad breath include the following:

Foods

The fact that food is the primary cause of bad breath is not a surprise to any of us. This is particularly valid for foods with potent aromas like onion and garlic. Another one of them is coffee. However, the bad odor these things cause is only momentary and will go away in a day or after brushing.

Your issue will be solved if you stay away from or consume fewer of these foods.

Smoking

If you have smoked for a while, you might have what is known as "the smoker's breath."

The nicotine and tar that have built up on the teeth and inside of the mouth are the source of this offensive smell.

You might believe that stopping smoking is the answer. But, no! Even though it can be reduced with good oral hygiene, that won't work the way you expect it to. Before you can finally be free of your bad breath issues, you will probably need to make several trips to the dentist.

Wet Mouth

If you've noticed, when you first wake up your breath isn't that pleasant. This is because we frequently experience dry mouth while we sleep. When your mouth is dry and not producing enough saliva to wash off the food particles, you can anticipate developing a bad breath problem because we need water and saliva to clean the mouth.

oral disease

When it comes to the main reasons why people get bad breath, this is ranked second. It is a gum ailment linked to bacterial infection. Deep spaces between your teeth and gums, known as periodontal pockets, are created as the issue worsens because the bone that supports your teeth is also damaged. Bacteria will be able to flourish in this situation. And as they consume the food particles trapped in these pockets, foul odor is also released, leading to bad breath. If a specific gum problem is the root of your bad breath issue, your dentist will be able to identify it.

Dental ailments and prosthetics

There is a high likelihood that you will have bad breath if you have decayed or abscessed teeth.

Dental professionals claim that any oral infection has a high likelihood of causing bad breath.

Full or partial dentures can both change how your breath smells.

These are merely a few of the causes of bad breath that you may experience. Another factor that can contribute to bad breath in a person is a sinus infection and other untreated medical conditions. In order to maintain constant fresh breath, you must also take care of your health.

Here some crucial bonus for you

1. Importance of Bad Breath Testers

For something ordinary, many do not understand fully what bad breath or halitosis isOr they might be aware of it but not fully understand why it happens.   Bad breath is not considered as a disease but this is where the problem lies. Many people don't consider it seriously, so that when it occurs they don't become aware that it has become their source of embarrassment to other people. If you don't want to be affected by the negative things that come with having bad breath, it is important that you are aware of the importance of bad breath testers.

A bad breath tester will not only allow you to learn if you are infected with such condition but will stop you from being the talk of the town because of this disgusting issue. The bad thing about halitosis is it is often impossible to conceal the reactions of the people you are talking with once they got the whiff of its nauseating smell. The reason is simply that, it is nauseating that it is hard for the people not to wince when your breath reaches their nostril. And if you are talking in close distance to someone, it is simply embarrassing and disturbing particularly if you witnessed how they made their face.

Bad breath testers will allow you to spot if you are a sufferer. This is the most important advantage why you should not ignore the fact that even if you are confident you don't have it, you need a bad breath tester. Many people suffer from halitosis but they are not aware of it. This is because one cannot easily smell their breath. It always takes someone for them to learn of the condition. It always has to be said to their face that there is something wrong with their dental hygiene because it is impossible to get whiff through your own nose.

But what if no one does that to you? What if all the people you encounter are just too embarrassed to tell you that there is something with your breath? And what if you are not conscious enough as to see the reason why they wince every time you speak so close with them? Now, that is a bad idea for these acquaintances will gradually get their distance from you. You don't want to be affected because of this turnout. You don't want to be emotionally and psychologically down because everyone seems to get their distance off you. These are all the more reason that you should consider bad breath testers an important part of your life.

The beauty of bad breath testers is that you don't have to have someone do it for you, which can be embarrassing at most times. You can test your breath at home and when you find out you are suffering from halitosis, you can do things that will solve your problem.

If the condition is not chronic, there are at home remedies and products over the counter which you can apply to yourself to cure it. But after doing these at home remedies and solutions and the halitosis persists, it is time for you to consult a medical professional for there might have something wrong with your medical condition.

It is either that you have some infections or you have some serious medical condition such as diabetes, kidney problems, and others, which can all cause your breath to become foul smelling.

2. Utilize Medicines for Bad Breath to Eliminate the Symptoms

You'll probably feel rejected if individuals run away from you when you try to strike up a discussion, thinking that they don't want you. This can be a terrible experience, especially if it occurs more than once, perhaps even more than twice. Instead of moping around, check yourself since you might have halitosis, or just foul breath. The truth is that most individuals find it intolerable when they smell someone else's foul breath.

It's funny how sometimes people can tolerate speaking with physically unclean people, but it is nearly impossible to continue a conversation with someone who exhales foul air. So, if you've been feeling rejected, ask yourself if you actually do have that feeling. If you do, don't complain about it; instead, look for bad breath remedies to treat it and prevent a repeat of the situation.

It's crucial to keep in mind that there are no miraculous drugs that will instantly cure your ailment when looking for bad breath remedies. First and foremost, you must identify the cause of your foul breath before purchasing an over-the-counter medication. There are medications for foul breath available, but they are actually provided in various ways. Not every one of these approaches is the best choice for your situation.

Therefore, identify the true cause of your halitosis before spending money on medications. There are many different causes of halitosis, and the one you have will largely determine how you should be treated.

So, for instance, if poor oral hygiene is the cause of your bad breath, all you need to do is make sure to remedy this mistake and keep up with it. But if your illness is more severe than that, you need to find another solution. For instance, before using bad breath medications, you must first treat the underlying medical disorders, such as sinusitis, tonsillitis, and others.

Meanwhile, severe foul breath symptoms can be treated with herbs, minerals, and other natural items. Many people have been depending on the wonders of natural resources because they not only efficiently treat problems with bad breath, but also because they include therapeutic natural chemicals that are perfect for promoting good physical condition and a healthy mouth. Depending on the true cause of your halitosis disease, additional types of bad breath medications may be suggested if you contact a dental professional or medical specialist.

No matter what anti-bad breath medications are recommended, it's crucial to maintain good dental hygiene in addition to taking the prescription. Among the most crucial good habits to adopt to prevent bad breath are brushing, flossing, mouthwashing, avoiding spicy foods, and taking care of your physical health.

Not only should you smile more frequently if your mouth and breath are in good health, but you should also feel more confident when speaking in front of an audience. You'll discover that it's also a quality that most people would prefer in a conversation partner rather than having to endure a terrible case of bad breath coming from the other person.

A good breath would never compromise with your social life, making it much easier and happier overall.

3. The Value of Understanding the Treatment for Bad Breath

Most people are fortunate to always have clean breath. These folks are fortunate in that they avoid having to deal with awkward situations when someone has to comment on how bad their breath is. However, not everyone is fortunate enough to avoid having terrible breath. In actuality, a lot of people have foul breath. And they are constantly searching for the greatest solution to their issues, which includes finding a cure for foul breath.

Knowing exactly what to do when you have bad breath and how to treat it is crucial if you truly want to have fresher breath once more. You can consult with your dentist about your issues. After all, your dentist is familiar with your dental history and will know the best course of action for you. On the other hand, you don't have to give up if you don't always feel at ease visiting the dental office.

Simply by practicing good dental hygiene, you may maintain fresh breath. when you can see, the waste products produced when the anaerobic oral bacteria feed inside our mouths are what generate bad breath. Therefore, according to specialists, you must ensure that you clean your mouth as thoroughly as you can in order to get rid of bad breath;

Remove food particles from the mouth where bacteria can feed on them. Reduce or eliminate the microorganisms that cause bad breath.

d. Maintain proper oral hygiene to prevent the growth of bacteria in your mouth.

Additionally, there are products that might minimize bad breath. The wisest course of action is still to do away with it. You'll regain your self-assured smile in this manner. Additionally, it's crucial to understand how to treat foul breath. Why? Well, because occasionally you might get foul breath, and if you don't know what the best treatment is, you might fear. On the other side, understanding what to do can enable you to resolve your issue effectively without experiencing anxiety or tension.

The three best remedies for bad breath are listed below:

1.) Watch What You Eat

Right, prevention is always preferable to treatment. As a result, you need to be aware that the different meals you eat have an impact on your breath. Anaerobic bacteria, according to studies, devour protein, and the consequence of their digestion is bad breath. This means that if you frequently consume protein-rich foods like meat and fish, you are probably going to have foul breath, especially if you don't properly clean your mouth. Now, if you typically consume more fruits and vegetables, you don't need to be concerned; just make sure to practice good mouth hygiene.

2.) Adequate Oral Care

• If you can't avoid eating meals high in protein, it's important to know how to properly brush your teeth. After eating, make sure to brush your teeth properly to avoid plaque building up on the teeth. On plaques, bacteria often grow. Additionally, flossing is crucial. You can use it to clean places your toothbrush can't.

3.) See the Documents

• Visiting a dentist is the best course of action if you believe that your bad breath issue is out of your control. In order to monitor your oral health, it is truly advised that you visit the dentist at least twice a year. Your dentist will be aware of the things to look for and how to treat your bad breath. Since gum diseases are among the most frequent causes of poor breath, a periodontal exam will almost certainly be performed. One of the things your dentist will do is remove any tartar if there is any.

4. Receive the Best Services for Bad Breath Treatment in Longmont!

Do you now reside in Longmont, Colorado? Do you struggle with your breathing and want the greatest remedy you can find? You know what, though? It should be simple to find foul breath treatment in Longmont because there are many dental offices and specialists in the area.

However, with so many choices available, it might be difficult to decide which clinic to go to. You wouldn't want to waste your hard-earned money on dental procedures that wouldn't yield fantastic results, would you?

Here are some suggestions if you're unsure of how to find the greatest dental care in Longmont:

• Request a referral. If you're seeking for reputable dental services, testimonials from your friends and family are excellent resources. You can ask them to suggest a dentist they are familiar with. You might get a trustworthy dental recommendation from your coworkers or even your family doctor. Ask your family dentist for a recommendation if you need to see a periodontist.

• Look up - if no one you know can recommend a reputable dentist, you can look one up on your own. Find licensed dentists in your region by conducting an online search. You might get a wonderful reference from your community dental society.

• You can also get in touch with a nearby dentistry school clinic.

• Verify the American Dental Association membership of the dentist you have in mind.

The suggestions listed above are just a few of the things you may do to identify a dentist who is reputable and trustworthy. Although having faith in people is not necessarily a bad thing, you should always exercise caution when it comes to your health.

You now need to be aware of the right dentist search techniques. Here are some pointers for finding a dentist in Longmont and getting treatment for foul breath:

• Verify that the dentist's office is easily accessible. You don't want to drive long distances merely to seek treatment for foul breath.

• Verify the cleanliness and organization of the dentist office. When treating a patient, make sure the dentist and his helpers are donning lab coats, masks, and gloves. Knowing how they sanitize their instruments and equipment is also a fantastic idea.

• Make sure to observe how the dentist and his employees deal with their patients. It's crucial that you feel at ease around them.

• You must also evaluate the dentist's proficiency; can he properly describe the issues and the solutions?